THE GENIUS GUIDE

to

PENIS PRIDE

THE GENIUS GUIDE

to

PENIS PRIDE

DICK JOHNSON

To order additional copies of this book, contact:
Xlibris
1-888-795-4274
www.Xlibris.com
Orders@Xlibris.com
787441

Contents

Chapter 1

About me

Sup? Allow me to introduce myself. My name is Dick Johnson, and I have a PhD. I know what you are thinking, no I am not a doctor. By PhD, I mean I have a pretty huge dick. It wasn't always that way as you will soon find out.

First, I would like to give you a whole hearted thank you for purchasing my book. You are now on your way to not only growing your penis, but also your all around self confidence. That is the reason I wrote this book. I am a professional coach in the art of penile enlargement, and also a mentor, life coach, and a friend. That is why I felt it was important to tell you a little bit about myself, and the story of how my friends began calling me "The Dick Man."

I grew up in a small town. I considered myself to me more of an awkward teenager. I spent most of my high school days being bullied and picked on. I was completely ashamed of my body....and most of all, my penis.

In my late teens, I discovered weight training. I loved doing exercises and watching my body transform. I noticed that over time, the muscles of the body could develop and change form. This is what got me thinking about penile growth. I knew that it had to be possible to grow my below average penis with the right techniques. I just didn't know how.

I did countless hours of research on penis growth, but what I found was a lot of bull shit quite honestly. I was determined to not let that stop me. So, what I did was, I started conducting experiments on myself! I would strongly recommend against this foolish idea, as I am very lucky that I did not cause any permanent damage to myself with my idiotic approach. Luckily for you, I have weeded out the dangerous part, and have figured out exactly what works, and what doesn't. Throughout my own experiments, I discovered a formula that worked for me. That's right. My penis got significantly longer, and thicker!

Now fast forward a few years to when I was in my 20's. I had become a very successful personal trainer. I loved helping people transform their bodies in the same way I had transformed my own. I knew what it was like to be out of shape and embarrassed, so my clients knew that I could relate to them. After several sessions with many of my male clients, they began to share their most intimate details with me. What I found was, a lot of them were suffering with the same problem that I had once suffered.

Under my direct guidance, I have helped over 50 men increase penile size and performance. That number continues to grow. By the time this book is published, my estimation is that this number will have doubled. That was my inspiration for writing this book. This is not a scam. I did not set out to make money from this. I am an honest man who truly cares about others, and I feel that nobody should have to be held back by having a penis that he is not happy with. It has now been over a decade since I began my journey toward penile enlargement. I feel that I have perfected the method at this point. I am willing to share my revolutionary method with the public. Thats just the kind of person I am. A man of the people.

Yours truly,
The Dick Man

Chapter 2

About the Book

First and foremost, you must understand that I am not a medical doctor, nor do I have any medical training. I am a normal man with first hand experience in the tried and true methods to penile enhancement, which I will explain in this book. The methods described in this book have not been backed by any scientific studies. However, there are many real world examples that have surpassed the expectations of penile advancement. The purpose of this book is not to sell any pill or potion, nor is it to sell any specific device. Things like that dont work anyways. What has been shown, time and time again, to add quality length and girth to the penis are the aformentioned techniques.

Obviously, there are no guarantees, but if you are looking to add quality gains to your member, you have come to the right place. I should know. I am not only the author of this book. I am also a former sufferer of what I call "small penis syndrome" or SPS. So if you suffer from SPS, or would just like to reap the benefit of an increase in size to your member, you have already conquered the first step by reading this book. Get ready to have a long dong....And if you already have one, get ready for it to be longer, and dongier.

Chapter 3

Does size matter?

A question when it comes to penis related debates is always the inevitable "does size really matter?" topic. In a simple word....Yes! Although allow me to explain why. Some people might argue, "Well, technically, a woman can give herself an orgasm with just one finger... Surely a finger is a lot smaller than an average penis...therefore, the size of the penis does not matter." This is absolutely correct, it is possible to give a woman an orgasm with a below average penis. Although if asked, every woman would prefer at least an average sized penis, even if she tells you she prefers small ones, she's lying. I do realize that a penis can become too big, at which point sex becomes painful, but thats a topic for a different debate.

Ok, lets get back to the topic. I want to use this space to describe why size matters for more personal reasons for a man. Having a large one will indeed improve your relationship and help you better satify your woman. We all know that. However, if your main objective for wanting a larger penis is solely to 'pick up more chicks' as they say, then I would advise you to stop reading now. You'd be much better off buying a book that teaches you how to make a million dollars, or teaches you how to be funny, or something else that women probably care more about than penis size. In our world, it's not as simple of an equation as big dicks equal tons of chicks. That is why before I give out my methods of penile growth, I want to be clear that this is all due to personal reasons, with the benefit of getting more ladies as an added bonus. Myself, and everyone else I have personally coached into having a package that they are proud of, have all done this for ourselves. The sense of accomplishment and pride that you get from having a penis that you're not ashamed of, is far more valuable than any amount of women that you could ever ask for. That's why if your wife or girlfriend sees you reading this book, you can assure her that you don't want to increase your manhood in order to cheat on her. Just say to her, "Baby, I'm doing this for me. And for us." That is why this book will be the most valuable tool you couldcever use for personal and relationship growth. In fact, I woudn't even consider this to be a sexual self help book, but rather an all around total body and mental self help. If you are ready to completely transform you life, not just your love life, let's get to it.

Chapter 4

The hand over hand tug

I thought it would be the most user friendly concept to start the techniques off with the most simple, yet very effective exercise for penile length. This practice has been used since the begining of time, and some users have boasted of gains of two or more inches in length just from this alone! The hand over hand tug can be done almost anywhere, at almost any time.

First, what you're going to want to do is make sure the area is nice and warm. Warmth opens up the veins, and enhances blood flow, allowing for oxygen, and nutrients to reach the area via blood flow. The shower would be an ideal spot to conduct this method, as a continual heat source is present... the water. However, it is not a technique that can only be conducted in the shower.

The next step in this method is to think of thoughts that will arouse you. The goal we are looking for here is for the penis to be engorged with as much blood as possible, without being fully erect. Some men refer to this penile state as having a "halfie," in other words, not an erection, but not quite flacid. When you feel as though you have achieved this state, and optimal blood flow is present, you are ready to begin.

Start at the base of the penis, and slowly stroke in a pulling motion from the base, through the shaft, and out the head of the penis. The hand should slide in one fluid motion. No lubrication is needed, however, it may be used if needed to enhance the experience. Once one hand has completed a "tug," the next hand should immediately follow, and so on, and so forth. The goal here is not to pull so hard as to cause discomfort, but to pull on it just enough to expand the connective tissue and penis muscles for growth. Ten minutes of performing this exercise during a five days on, two days off regimine seems to be the most effective manner for the body to take full advantage of the hand over hand tug.

I cannot stress enough the importance of visualization in this, and any other methods included in this book. I firmly believe in a saying that goes "you have to think big to grow big." I will discuss this more in a later chapter, but in the example of the hand over hand tug, you should visualize that your penis is a neverending, long rope that is all tucked inside your body. Now with every tug, you keep pulling more and more of this rope out from within yourself. As you pull, the rope gets longer and longer. The penis will expand and grow, and the only limitation for the growth is what the mind limits itself to. Please refer to the images to get a better idea of this technique, as well as all of the other ones included in this book.

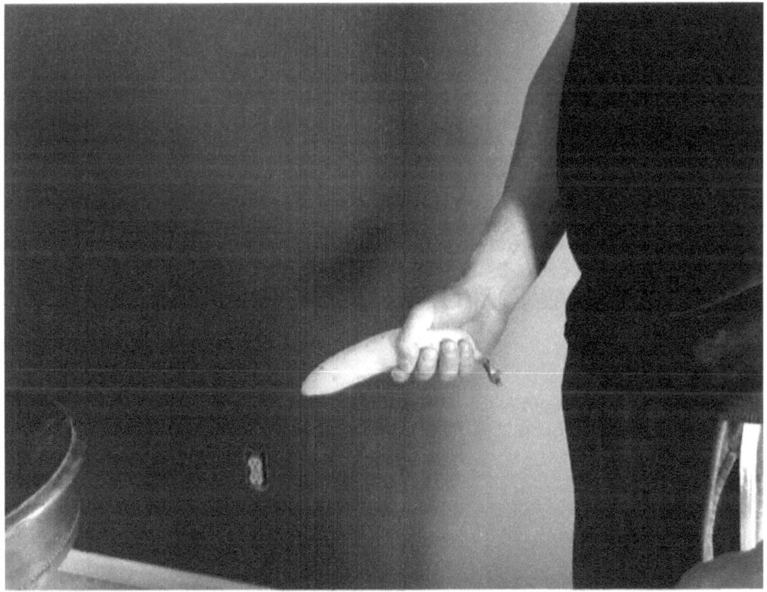

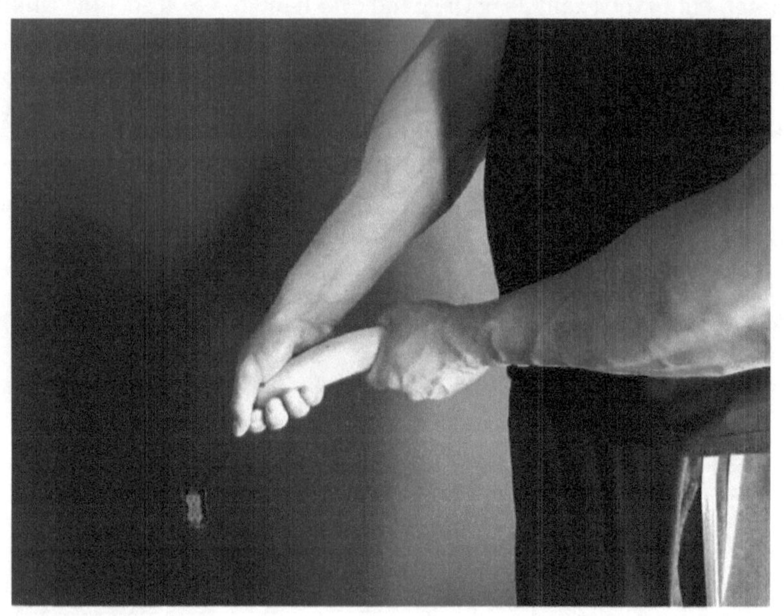

Chapter 5

The squeeze and stretch

This is a technique that I hold near and dear to my heart. Out of all the techniques detailed in this book, this one stands out as my personal favorite. The squeeze and stretch is a fairly simple maneuver to perform, however, it involves complete concentration. If performend correctly, the squeeze and stretch can be extremely effective, and i can attest to that.

To fully understand this technique, we must first examine the anatomy of the penis. The penis is composed of a major muscle called the bulbospongiosus muscle. Without getting too scientific and boring, this muscle contributes to erections, ejaculation, and the sensation of having an orgasm. Obviously, this is an extremely important muscle to any male who wants to get the most out of his sexual experience.

The theory behind the squeeze and stretch is to target the bulbospongiosus muscle, and train it, causing hypertrophy. In layman's terms, hypertrophy means growth, so in essence, we are going to grow the muscle of the penis. This is very similar to when a bodybuilder goes to the gym and performs exercises to make the biceps, or any other muscle grow. The same can be done for the muscles of the penis, once the technique is mastered that is.

To begin, visualize that you are in the middle of urination. Your urine is flowing strongly out of your penis. Now, imagine that you must abruptly stop urinating. Squeeze the muscles of your penis to fight back the urine from exiting the penis. Once you have felt the muscles of your penis contract, hold this contraction and slowly count to ten. Be patient, as not everybody will master this squeeze on the first attempt. After your have held your squeeze for your ten count, immediately relax the muscles of your penis, and using your index finger and thumb, gently pull the penis by its head away from your body to achieve a stretch. As in the previous chapter, our objetive here is not to pull the penis so hard as to cause discomfort. The goal is to simply achieve a stretch, much like you would do to any other muscle in the body before or after any exercise. Once you have performed a squeeze for a ten count, followed by a stretch for another ten count, you have completed one repetition. An effective reime to maximize hypertrophy of the bulbospongiosis muscle is 10-15 repetitions of the squeeze and stretch, performed daily.

The main focus of this book is to discuss penile enlargement, but the squeeze and stretch may offer many other sexual benefits. Men who often partake in the practice of the squeeze and stretch find that they have fewer problems with erectile dysfunction, premature ejaculation, and report to have fuller feeling erections. This makes sense, because as the muscle grows and gets stronger, the body becomes more in control of the penis. So incorporate the squeeze and stretch into your penile regime, and you too may experience the growth, and many other benefits.

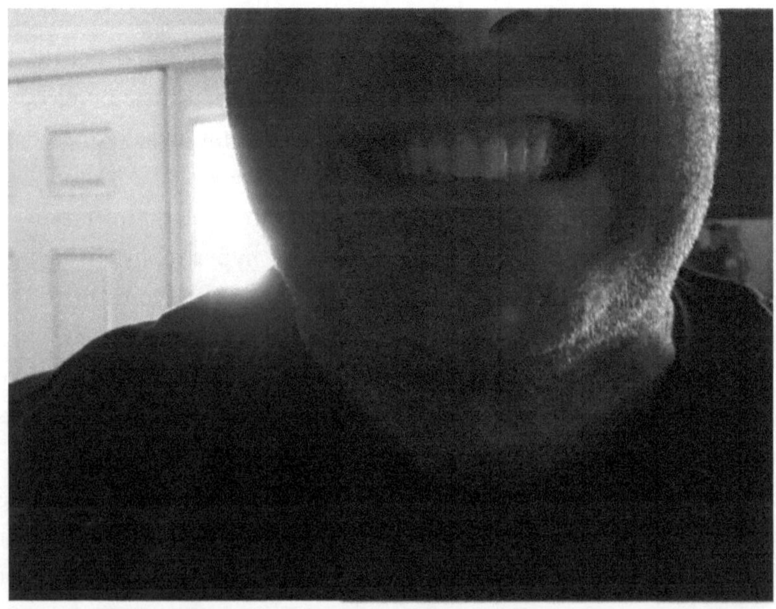

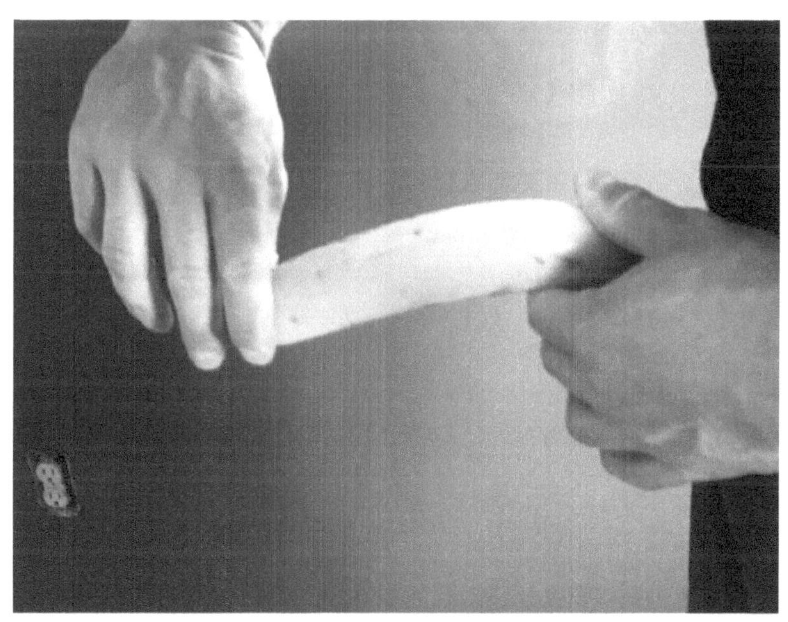

Chapter 6

Jelqing

Anyone who has done a good bit of research on the topic of penile enhancement has no doubt heard of the practice of jelqing. This is a practice that dates back many years, and is believed to have roots in the Middle East. The practice of jelqing is very controversial, which is why I almost did not include it in this book. However, I do believe that if used properly, jelqing can be an effective way to lengthen the penis. Through my groundbreaking research, I have perfected this art.

So, for those who don't know I'll explain what is jelqing and how to jelq. Jelqing (pronounced Jel-King) is basically a series of stretching and pusing the penis at the head to force blood to the head of the penis and not let it out from there. This, in theory, will cause the penis to expand. The penis is squeezed at the base using the thumb and index finger, then these fingers and slid to the head of the penis, and held in this area for a matter of time. The process is repeated over and over.

So why is this controverial? Well, the thing I don't like about this practice is, there are several idiots online making false claims about this practice. These people, who have not studied anything about penile enhancement, are saying ways to improve your jelqing to make it more effective. Remember, if you didn't hear it from me, The Dick Man, it probably isn't true.

The first thing you want to never do is to jelq an erect penis, or one that is close to being erect. I tell all of my clients to never practice jelqing on a penis that is more than 50% engorged with blood. Any more erect that that, and you can actually damage the penile tissue, and in some cases could even lead to erectile dysfunction. So when people online claim that jelqing an erection is a new, innovative way to grow your penis...Do not believe them!

The next bit of misinformation when it comes to the art of jelqing, is that the squeeze at the head should be held for a longer period of time to yield better results. This is a completely false statement. The slide from the base to the head is JUST as important as the squeeze at the head of the penis. So, I would recommend a squeeze of approximately two seconds on the head. You do not want to squeeze your penis to death.

Also, so called "experts" would like you to believe that the more you jelq, the more results you will obtain. Very untrue. Jelqing is a technique that we want to be very careful not to overdo. Anything more than ten minutes of jelqing is counter productive. Rest days from jelqing are also just as important as jelq days, so make sure you give that penis a break. Start out with an every other day regiment, and go from there, but be sure to never exceed 5 days of jelqing per week.

I have no problem with the Middle East, but they do not have the best track record when it comes to penile practices to say the least. That is why much caution should be used with jelqing, as well as any other technique that originates from this part of the world. Remember, this is the same place that came up with taqaandan, which is the practice of basically breaking your penis in half to hear a popping sound. I will discuss this more in a later chapter. However, if done properly, as outlined above, jelqing can be an effective means of lenghtening the penis. It is very important to proceed with caution, and not to stray away from the protocol that is listed in this chapter. I was coined the nickname "Dick Man" for a reason. It's because I care about you and your penis. So if anyone tries to tell you that they know of a better form of jelqing or any other practice mentioned in this book, Do Not Listen!

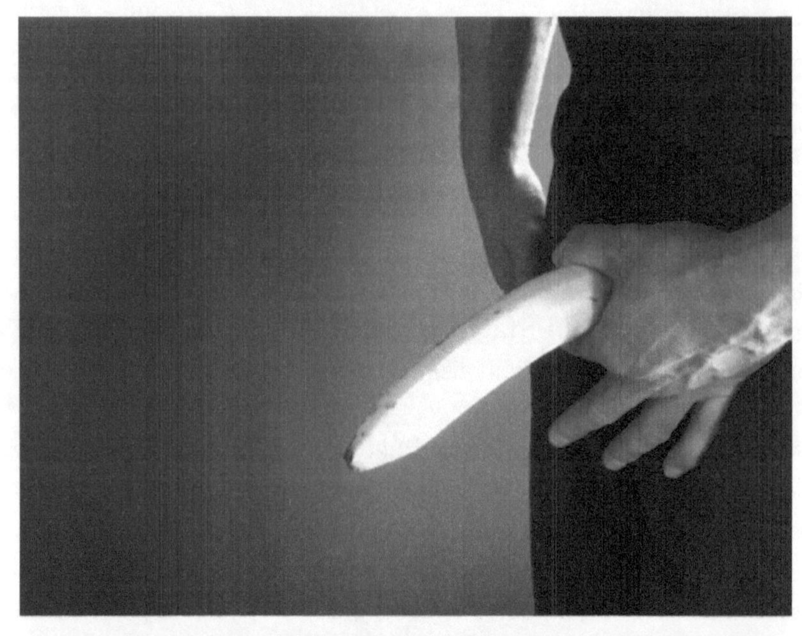

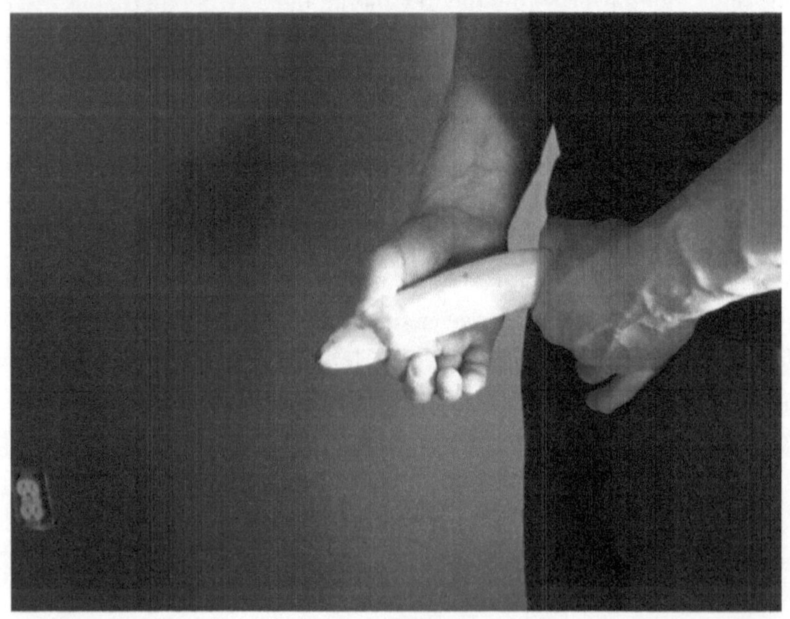

Chapter 7

The mummy

If you're anything like me, then it probably feels like your penis has a mind of its own. Sometimes, the thing feels like it's at its full potential. Other times... ehhhh not so much. This is a problem I struggled with for years. Depending on what mood you caught me in, my penis size would be affected. In fact, the effect of my mood on my penis was so dramatic, that sometimes I wondered if it was even my dick or somebody else's. This became very annoying, because I never knew from one minute to the next whether my penis would be normal, or shriveled up.

Now when I talk about this, notice that I will use the word was. My penis WAS a problem for me for a lot of years. Fortunately, I have developed a method to correct this issue. There are some changes in penis size that are unavoidable, for instance the "shrinkage" experienced due to cold temperatures. This happens because the penis needs to get closer to the body to protect itself and the semen from the cold weather. In this chapter, I'm talking about the fluctuations in size that are caused by changes in the mood, and are completely fixable.

Although sometimes it might seem that men think using their penises, the penis is actually controlled by the mind, and doesnt actually have a mind of its own. If I've said it once, I've said it a hundred times, there is a direct connection between the brain and the penis. Mood and state of mind can definitely explain why the penis seems to alter its size throughout the day. Think about it, when you are aroused, the penis becomes affected by your arousal, and gets bigger. Your body is in an altered state, the state of arousal. Now lets look at the opposite end of the spectrum. When the man is in an altered state that is opposite from the state of arousal, such as anger, nervousness, or any other unpleasant state, then the penis is also in that altered state. So, what do you think happens to the penis? That's right. This is the body's natural response. For example, the muscles of the abdomen tense up and contract to prepare for impact if the mind senses that a person is about to get punched in the gut. It's this same adrenaline rush that causes the penis to shrink when the mental state is altered. This explains why if you've ever gone to show your penis to someone, all of a sudden it becomes half of its normal size. While we are glad that our abdominal muscles tense up as a response to the adrenaline rush in the example above, we would like to train our penises to not shrink as a result of this same adrenaline spike.

So let's get down to business. How did I train my penis to not respond to fear, anger, or nervousness? Well, behaviors that are ingrained into our bodies take time to break, but it is certainly possible. All you have to do is not allow the penis to shrink due to these situations, and eventually the penis will learn not to shrink on its own. And we do this by applying a device that you can do on your own, in a process that I like to call "penis mummification."

To start this procedure, take a tissue, paper towel, or piece of toilet paper, you get the message. Wrap the tissue around the shaft of the penis, covering the base to the head, but keep the head free. Next, you will need masking tape. Make sure that you are using masking tape and not a stronger tape that will be too tight and reduce the blood flow to the penis. Wrap the tape around the shaft, starting from the base and working your way up, again leaving the head free. Do not wrap the tape so tight that you can feel your pulse in your penis. We are going for a nice, comfortable, snug fit. This should be worn for the entire day, so make sure that you aren't in a position that someone will have to see your penis, if you are the type of person that wants to keep this all a secret. A great idea is to wrap your penis up before you go to work, and then comfortably leave your wrap on all day while you are at work. Chances are, you will forget it is even there, and just go about your daily activities as normal. The penis, however, won't forget that *it is mummified. When the mind feels these altered states which we have discussed earlier, the penis will not be able to contract and shrink, because the wrap and tape will keep it elongated, preventing it from shrinking. After several days of this practice, the penis will be trained to not respond to the body's adrenaline spike, and it will stay in its natural, full state. Each person's response time to this technique is going to be different, so don't feel upset if your buddy can train his penis quicker than yours. This technique, as well as all other techniques will not produce overnight results. Remember, this is a marathon and not a sprint. The practice of penis mummification, I can tell you has completely changed my life, and I know it will change yours. Don't let your mind be an enemy to your penis anymore. Turn your emotions into your best friend. Start mummifying your penis today.

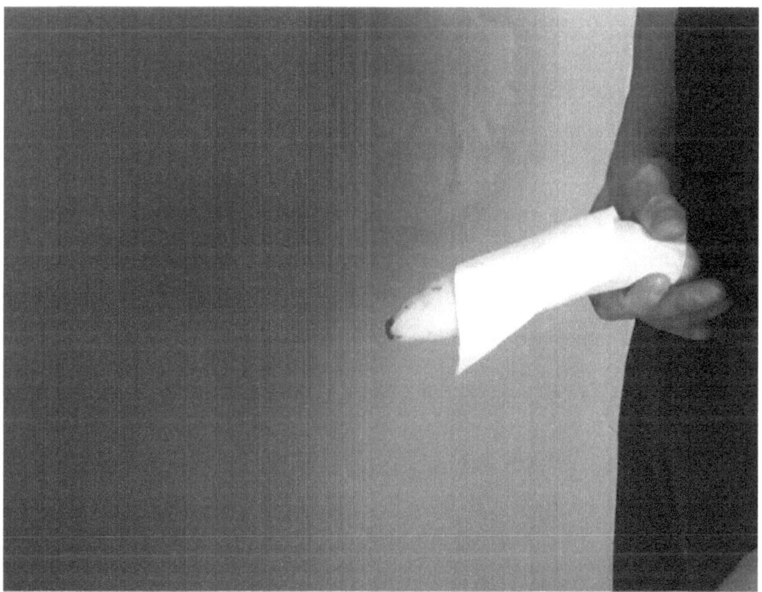

Chapter 8

Visualize

In my last chapter, and in various other parts of this book, I've discussed in great detail the importance of the mind in connection with your penis. In this chapter, I would like to follow up on all of that and really hammer home these points. This is very crucial to understanding this book, and getting the most out of it.

Did you ever go through a bad break up, or maybe a fight with your partner, and she told you in anger that you have a small penis? I have. And you know what? For several weeks after that, my penis actually did seem smaller to me. If the mind can make your penis seem smaller, it would only reason to conclude that the opposite would also be true. Could surrounding ourselves with positive people who tell us that it is huge actually make it bigger?

Let me tell you something about the power of the mind. I have heard stories, maybe you have heard them too, for example, a person gets diagnosed with some terrible disease. You may have heard of people who lose the will to live because of their situation, and the person ends up dying. You may have also heard about people who decide they are going to win this battle, and fight, and they survive their ailments.

I heard a story of one of these fighters who refused to give up on life and let the disease kill him. Every day this person would visualize his white blood cells attacking the bad cells in his body. He imagined his body getting stronger and the disease getting weaker. He visualized himself as powerful, and the disease as weak. Do you want to know what happened to this man with the disease? He beat it. He conquered his disease because he had the mental toughness to beat it. If a person wants to win, they might. Doctors have stated that if they told all of their healthy patients that they only had one year to live...a large percentage of those people actually would die within that year. These are people with nothing wrong with them. So, what does this tell us? It tells us that if a person believes in something, it can become a reality.

My guess is you know where I am going with this. And honestly, why shouldn't I go here with it. Do you see how this makes perfect sense. Do you understand that maybe you are limiting your penis right now because you are ashamed of it? Here is what I want you to do. Every night as you lay in bed, I want you to visualize your penis growing. Don't fill your head with any negative thoughts. Envision your penis growing larger and larger. Visualize the blood filling up your penis and allowing it to expand. Each day I want you to imagine that your unit is so big that it barely fits in your pants. And dont just think about it. Believe it. Feel your penis halfway down your leg, rubbing against your thigh. Don't limit your penis size to what your mind says it is. If the mind says it is huge, the body will follow. From now on, only refer to your penis by terms that imply bigness and size such as shlong, dong, unit, enforcer, mandingo, anaconda. Don't refer to it by terms that make it seem small, like willy, jimmy, shawty, pee pee, wee wee, or prick.

I'm not trying to tell you to be in denial about your penis. In fact, by purchasing this book, it shows that you have come to terms with the problem, and are ready to do something about it. This is more about positive imagery and visualization about your penis. And most importantly, never feel inadequate because of your penis. Just realize that there is plenty of room for growth, growth can be possible, and know that whether or not you can get it to grow, it has no bearing on your manliness or who you are as a person. Continue to meditate on this and you will come to realize that you have a new outlook on life.

Chapter 9

Masturbate your way to a bigger penis

At this point, you should already know the benefits of using your penis for sexual arousal. If you are fortunate enough to have the opportunity to have sex, by all means, I would suggest that you take full advantage of it. Eliminating excess sperm is optimal for the overall penis health and function. However, if you are like the majority of men, and do not have access to sex at all times, then the alternative option is self pleasure, in other words, masturbation. The frequency of masturbation should depend on each man. Everybody is different. More often is optimal, but I am hesitant to suggest a frequent regimen due to the fact that many men can become addicted to masturbation, and this can really cause a slew of problems. If I may make a suggestion, I would recommend self pleasure as often as possible, without it being allowed to consume your life. You will know how much is too much, and how much is the right amount.

Now on to the good part. You might already know how sex with another person can improve the quality of your sex life, but you might be wondering if having sex with yourself can also play a part. Well the simple answer is Yes! Of course, it's not just as easy as that though. I am going to lay out a simple trick that will maximize your alone time, and take it to a new level.

During a normal masturbation session, most men achieve climax by grabbing a firm grip around the penis, with or without lube, and stroking it back and forth. The problem with this procedure, is that every time the man completes the stroke toward his body, he is compressing the tedons and tissues of the penis. This actually can train your penis not to grow. Remember, even though normal masturbation mimicks the motion of sexual intercourse, it is very different because during sex, the orifice is not grabbing a hold of the penis and forcing it closer to the body.

I would like to teach you my secret to masturbating to increase the size of your penis. You will find this method to be effective and enjoyable. In fact, every man i have introduced this method to claims to prefer it to their old way of masturbating. This task is easier accomplished using lubrication. Although not required, it is highly suggested. Any form of lubrication will do the trick. It doesn't have to be some type of fancy store bought product. Begin this method by taking a firm grip at the base of your penis using your thumb and index finger only. This grip should hold back the excess skin of the erect penis. At this point, the head of the penis should begin to swell as it engorges with bood. Next, using the hand that is free, apply lubrication to the erect penis. Maintain the grip on the base of the penis. With the hand not gripping the base of the penis, use your fingertips to gently stroke the penis in the direction away from the body. The hand should move in one fluid motion, gently sliding the fingertips from the base of the penis toward the tip until ejaculation is completed.

The reason that this motion is so effective is beacuse it works with the body's natural rhythmic pulses. This is how masturbation was intended before the modern man put his own twist on it. This practice might feel a bit different at first, but after getting used to it and getting the hang of it, you will realize that it is enjoyable, and you will start to notice a differece in the quality of the firmness of your erections, and also, the size of your erections.

Chapter 10

Belt method

The next installment of this book is based off of a practice which dates back thousands of years. This practice has been used by the Kayan tribes since the first century, or possibly before. I am sure you have seen it at one time or another throughout your life. Women of the Kayan tribes can be spoted and identified by their long necks, sometimes reaching 11 inches! You might be asking, "Well thats fascinating and all, but how in the world does this relate to penile growth?" Well, allow me to explain.

The neck of the Kayan women is placed inside metal rings. Over time, more and more rings are added to the neck, causing the neck to grow taller and longer, giving these women an almost giraffe type of appearance. If we examine this practice scientifically, we can conclude that what is really happening with this processs is actually different than what we think. As more metal is wrapped around the neck, the shoulders of the Kayan woman get pushed down. This happens little by little, as to not cause severe pain all at once. Its more of a gradual thing. In actuality, the neck only "grows" because the shoulders go down. The head doesn't actually go up. This is a very important concept to understand. The necks of these women get bigger, because another body part of theirs got pushed away.

How does this concept apply to penile growth? Am I suggesting that we all wrap a bunch of rings around our peckers to force the body away from our dicks and push it out farther? Absolutely not! However, there is a very simple, yet effective method to achieve the same result as the neck growth, only on a smaller scale in the penile area. This is simply by pushing the area directly above the penis a little bit back. This area, you might have been heard as referred to as the FUPA....which stands for Fat Upper Penis Area. Even if you don't have much fat there, you can still benefit from this area being pushed back.

Keep in mind, this is a slow process that over time could yield fantastic results. Just like the Kayan women, we can grow our members steadily, day by day. As this is an every day process, it is important to complete this as much as possible.

What you will need for this task is a simple, ordinary belt. Any belt will do, but i find that a more wide, sturdy belt works the best. This belt will be wrapped around the waist, just above the base of the penis, and over top the the underwear, but underneath the pants. This way, nobody will know that it is there. You will want to tighten the belt as tight as you can so that it is still comfortable, but doesn't cut off the circulation. The muscles should feel tight underneath the belt, and the lower abdomen should feel slightly sucked in. You are now able to comfortably go about your day, while at the same time adding the important size to your penis.

As with the Kayan women, the key to this method is to gradually increase the pressure over time. You will notice that after several days of wearing your belt at the same tightness, you will be able to handle more, and can make it tighter. As long as it doesnt cause any discomfort, you can go ahead and tighten the belt as you feel able to. Over time, the pelvic area will become more drawn in, like a vaccuum effect, thus lenghthening the penis, and allowing for further penetration.

Chapter 11

Pulsation

Before I start this chapter, I want to clear up some of the negative feedback about penile enlargement. Many men, probably who have either given up on trying to get a bigger penis, or do not want anyone else to have a bigger one, are out there saying that it is impossible to change the penis. Allow me to give examples of why I believe that these people are wrong. The first example is the number of men who have formerly had a natural, slight curve to the penis. It could be either to the left or right. This is a simple fix for anyone looking to straighten it out. When a man who has a bend in his penis forces the penis in the opposite direction every time it hangs, eventually over time, it will straighten out. Thats one example of a penis changing. Another example I'd like to present is when a man always uses the same hand each time that he masturbates. These men have actually come to me and complained about how the penis favors one side or the other, by having a type of lean or twist in the direction of the hand that always gets used for self pleasure. If it is possible to change the penis is this way, it shows that the penis is extremely changeable. It's not some type of organ that is unchangeable. Therefore, it's no stretch of the imagination to conceive that if the penis is proven to be changeable, then size is certainly something that can change. This is the principle that our next exercise revolves around.

As we continue this book, the tasks may seem to get more complicated involving growth of the penis. The pulsation method may seem complicated at first, but as with many things in life, the things that are more complicated, can often times be more effective. This exercise is a safe and effective exercise, in my opinion, to add extreme length and crazy girth to the penis.

The pulsation method is one of the only times that I say an erect penis should be used. Due to this fact, obviously it is highly recommended that this exercise is performed in complete privacy. I am not responsible for anyone's actions regarding sexual harrassment. Once you have achieved an erection, the next thing you will need to do is feel for your pulse. You can check your pulse on your wrist, below where the thumb connects, or on the artery on the side of your neck. You do not need to count your heart rate or anything. Just feel for the rhythm of your heart beat. The idea here is to detect the pattern of your heart rate, so that you will know each time your heart beats, even before it beats. For example, my heart is currently beating now...now...now...now...now...now.

After you have found the rhythm of your heart rate, you are ready to begi the technique. Place both of your hands on your erect penis. One hand should be placed at the very base of the penis, and the other hand should be placed directly above that hand. Don't worry if there is overlap of your hands. Even the largest of dicks have overlap. If you can only get one hand around it, thats ok too. Just put the other one on top of that hand. Eventually, you might be able to get both of them comfortably around the penis.

With the hands now wrapped around your erect penis, you are now going to mimic the heart beat by squeezing the penis with both hands at the same time as your heart beats. As the heart muscle relaxes, your hands too shall relax. So, each squeeze should only last a fraction of a second.... the time it takes for the heart to beat. For example. If my heart is beating now...now...now...now...now, I am going to squeeze my penis now...now... now...now...now. It is this repeated jolt in which allows the erect penis to become more full, and work toward optimal growth. Again, the goal here is not to squeeze so hard as to cause pain. We are simply looking to put a little pressure in there. Both hands should squeeze simultaneously, in unison with the heart beat. This can be done everyday, for about ten minutes.

The reason why I feel that pulsation is essential for maximizing your penile growth is because you are allowing the hands and heart muscle to work as one to zone in and target the area needed for growth. It also helps the mind to become more in touch with the heart rate, as well as the penis. Remember, your mind is in control of your penis.

As the heart pumps, it is rushing blood to various blood vessels and arteries throughout the body...including the penis. By adding the extra squeeze to assist with the blood flow, the vessels of the penis can expand and push against the wall of the penis, opening up this area for some intense growth. This exercise is only for men who are serious about their penile enlargement.

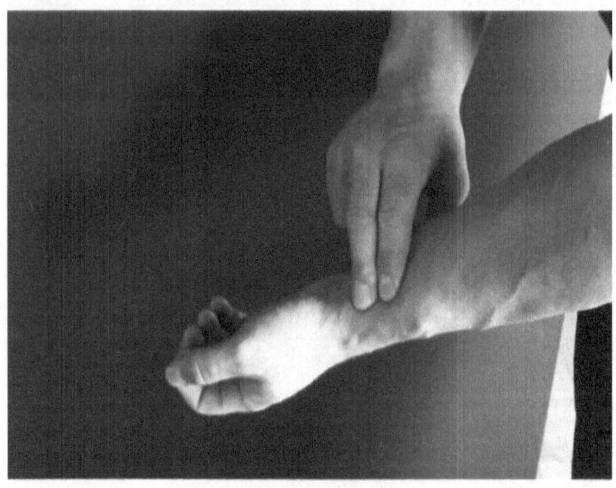

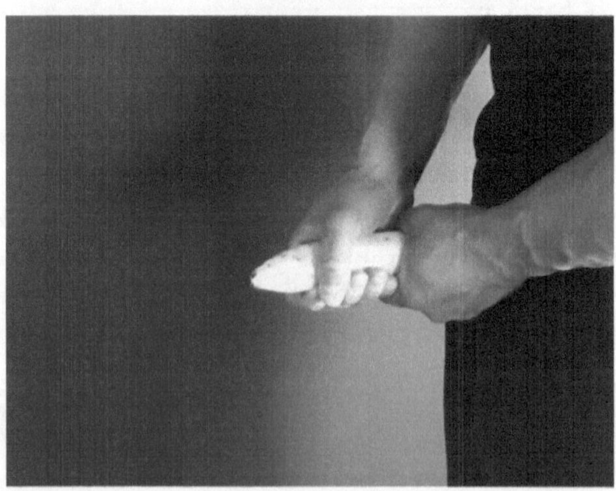

Chapter 12

If you don't use it, you lose it.
If you do use it, it'll grow!

This is a topic that gets touched on many times throughout this book. That is why I wanted to just take a minute here to write a quick passage about how using your penis can help it to grow. It is something that can't be stressed enough, that's why i dedicated a short chapter just for this topic. I wanted to make sure that you don't forget it. Any man who has seen tv shows, or participated in "guy talk" has heard of the phrase at one time or another "If you don't use it, you lose it." It might sound like an old wives tale, but believe it or not, there is some truth to this statement. Think about it. When a person wakes up after an extended period of time being in a coma, that person cannot walk, or even function. This is because the muscles in the legs have shrunk and weakened to a point where they are not usable. The person has to retrain him or herself in order to walk again. This loss in muscle strength is referred to as atrophy. So if this happens to the muscles of the legs, and we have already pointed out earlier in the book that the penis contains a muscle, what do you think will happen to that muscle if it is not used?

Now on the other hand, lets consider the opposite end of the spectrum. If a person goes to the gym everyday and exercises their legs, the legs will adapt to the training by getting stronger and growing. So if you don't use the legs, you lose them, but if you do use them, they grow. Have you ever heard the penis called a third leg? Do you think that is just a coincidence? I think not. The same concept that gets applied to the legs can also be applied to the penis. You will realize that much of the topics I discuss in this book make perfect sense. You are probably even thinking, "Hmmmmm, I never thought about it like that." Thats why this isn't rocket science, but it is in a way very clear cut. That is basically all I need to say about this topic. I just want you to be aware that you need to use your penis. Try to get an erection as many times as possible throughout the day. Make a game of it. You don't have to complete the task and have an orgasm. Just pop a nice boner here and there. It'll be great fun and if will keep that thing from atrophy.

Chapter 13

Sleep trick

What if there was a way to increase the size of your package, just by doing something you are already doing every night? Sleeping! In this chapter, I would like to discuss the importance of sleep for penile growth, and how we can optimize it to actually grow our member as we sleep.

Any weightlifter or athlete will tell you that the best way to recover from hard exercise is to get a good night's rest. Most experts recommend eight hours of sleep per night. Your mother probably told you when you were little that if you get to bed early and get a good night's sleep, you will grow up to be big and strong. So, sleep has always been associated with growth since the beginning of time. How then, can we use this weapon to maximize our penis growth? This is a simple trick that I will explain.

When any exercise is performed to any muscle group, penis included, the muscle and tissue gets broken down by the body. The way that the muscle grows is during the rest period. The body actually rebuilds the fibers that were broken down during exercise, and rebuilds them bigger than they were before. By performing the techniques demonstrated in this book, followed by the sleeping technique that I will describe, you body will be primed to kick the penile growth into second gear.

When we are sleeping, we want to be extra careful to not restrict the penis by wearing tight underwear or shorts. Briefs are just about the worst item you can wear if you are looking to optimize penile growth. Now,

I know that certain times in life, it could be unavoidable to wear brief type underwear, but there is never a time that briefs should be worn to bed. Never never never. A lose fitting boxer short would be a much better option, and sleeping naked would be better yet. However, I have developed a method that beats even sleeping naked when it comes to the topic.

For this practice, which has been effective for my own penis enhancement journey, you will need a night pair of shorts possibly made out of spandex or some type of stretchy material. Don't worry, I am not contradicting my previous statements about tight shorts. You will see where I am going with this. Next, you will cut a circular hole in those shorts with a scissors, and make that hole big enough for your penis and your testicles to fit through. The hole should be made directly where the penis and testicles would naturally hang. Don't make the hole too big or too small. If the hole is too big, it will defeat the purpose. If it is too small, it will cut off the circulation. Just a nice comfortable hole to put your dick and balls out. As each man's endowment is different, I cannot give an exact circumference of the hole, but roughly the size of a tennis ball should be a good starting point. Simply place the penis and testicles outside of the hole, and sleep as normal.

The reason that I find this technique to be so effective is because of something called blood flow occlusion. This is basically a term for restricted blood flow. The shorts are not so tight that they stop the circulation of blood flow to the legs and feet, but they do compress the legs slightly. Just enough to funnel the blood into the area that isnt covered by the shorts, the penis. As the heart rushes blood into the limbs of the body, these special shorts help to direct the blood flow into the area where we want it the most for growth. This works very much is the same way any other type of funnel works. It disburses the liquid into a single, targeted area. The more blood we get into the penis, the more it feels alive. The more it becomes stimulated by our blood. This will help the natural, nocturnal erections. So, don't be surprised if you start waking up will a full, hard penis after starting this technique. Use this every night when you sleep, in conjunction with the other great exercises contained in this book. Your penis will thank you.

Chapter 14

Debunking the pill myth

By now, I'm sure you've heard of the many over the counter pills, drinks, and creams which promis to enlarge the penis. Perhaps you've even tried some of these for yourself. Maybe you've seen the commercials on t.v. and they were so inticing, that you couldn't help but fall for this snake oil scam. The penis enlargement pill industry has become a multi-million dollar industry, lining the pockets of the makers of these pills and potions. The problem is, that's about all these pills do, put money in the pockets of their creators. You may be thinking, "but Dick Man, I, or somebody I know, has taken these pills and gotten results." Let me explain why they think they have gotten results.

The human penis is composed mostly of spongy tillue filled with blood vessels. There is no pill or cream that can make a bodily tissue grow, and to think that it could be possible is just plain wrong. The reason why some people feel that they have had positive results from these pills is because the pills contain ingredients that help the body to produce nitric oxide, which aids in blood flow, and that can allow the penile tissue to be filled with blood. Now, am I suggesting that it is a bad thing to fill the penis with blood? Absolutely not! In fact, several times throughout this book, I encourage it. And I also encourage as many erections as possible throughout the day. And we all know that an erection is just when the penis is filled up with blood.

The purpose of this chapter is not to deter men from using suplementation to increase blood flow to the penis. In a later chapter, I will even discuss supplements that will help to optimize blood flow to the penis. The point I am making here is this. These penile enlargement pills typically go for about $100 per bottle. A bottle is only a month or so supply. So basically, you are spending a huge amount of money for a product that is, at best, a combination of things that you could buy for a fraction of that price. The techniques in this book will far surpass any pill or cream that you can buy.

Think about it. A pill that you take through your mouth, that somehow targets one one specific appendage of your body and makes it grow? Clearly this is too far fetched to be true. A cream that you rub on makes slightly more sense, but still falls short in actually producing the type of growth we are looking for. So stop giving your money to these companies who promise results but never live up to their expectations.

Chapter 15

Diet and Supplementation

As stated in the previous chapter, as well as several other times throughout this book, blood flow is essential for the maintenance of healthy penile function and growth. Indeed, blood flow is an important factor that can never be neglected. Without a healthy flow of blood to the penis, all of the oxygen and nutrients cannot reach the area of the body that needs them the most. Remember, blood caries the healthy rejuvinating ingredients in order to repair and expand. So, let's delve into ways that we can utilize our eating habits to capitalize on this very important factor in penile enlargement.

Omega 3 fats-

Unless you've been living under a rock, chances are you have heard of this type of fat. These are mostly present in fish, and certain type of nuts i.e. flax seeds. Entire books can be written on the health benefits of this type of fats, however, for the purposes of this topic, I will explain how omega 3's can allow more blood flow to where we want it the most... our Johnson. First of all, studies have shown the great benefits of omega 3's in fighting cholesterol build up. Think about this. If cholesterol is built up around the blood vessels and arteries, that means there is less room for blood to pass through those vessels and arteries. If blood can't pass through, how can we expect this blood to get to our penis? I have this saying that goes, "a healthy heart, is a healthy penis." Omega 3's also reduce inflammation in the body which also helps blood get to the dick. Also, omega 3's thin the blood out, helping it to pass right along to down town if you know what I mean. Surely, omega 3's pack a thunder punch when it comes to penile enlargement. Make sure to eat wild caught fish every day, or take omega 3's in pill for which is probably easiest.

Red Wine-

Ok, you might be thinking, what kind of book advises the use of alcohol? Well, of course I am only advocating responsible use, never in excess, and never drink and drive. However, when consumed responsibly, the antioxidants and resveratrol in red wine are great for your blood pressure and blood flow. The blood thinning properties of the red wine also help to make it a fantastic beverage with dinner that might help to grow your penis. A staple in the Mediteanean diet is to drink red wine. I wonder if any studies have been done on the men who follow this diet, and the size of their dicks... if any scientists are out there, please look into this.

Vitamin C-

The reason I included vitamin C, well there are several reasons. We all know that this vitamin does wonders for the immune system, keeping the body healthy. One could stipulate that the peis is part of the body, so a healthy body is a healthy penis. I also need to point out that vitamin C plays a key role in circulation. Vitamin C helps with the capillaries that carry blood from the arteries to the cells. Without getting too scientific on you, just take my word for it that foods high in this vitamin are healthy for you, and good for you know what.

Garlic-

Here's a fun one. We all know that garlic and wreak havoc on your breath. What can garlic do for your penis? Will, quite simply, it can do much for it. Garlic is great for lowering blood pressure, which I already touched on is great for maximum penis. Garlic also helps to dialate the arteries, or expand them if you will. These arteries open up and let that blood surge into the right place. I recommend eating garlic raw, as heating it up can inhibit some of its great benefits. You can also find it in pill form for those of you who dont like the flavor.

Beets-

Remember last chapter when I talked about nitric oxide? Well, this vegetable has been shown to actually increase nitric oxide levels in the body. Nitric oxide is the substance for gym rats that "pumps you up." Nitric oxide opens up the arteries better than any other substance. The way beets increase nitric oxide is because they contain nitrate. When it is ingested, the body converts nitrate into nitric oxide. The nitric oxide opens up the veins. The open veins allow the blood to flow. The blood flows to the dick. The dick grows. Success. It is simple philosophy 101. Some great amino acids you can take to increase you nitric oxide levels in the body are L-arginine, as well as L-citrulline.

Now I want to mention a few foods to avoid-

Salt in excess- We all know that salt can make some things taste better. We also all know that there are a lot of health risks associated with eating an excessive amount of salt in our diet. I'm sure you've learned somewhere, whether from school, or your doctor, that salt is rough on heart pressure. I don't think I need to say anything else about eating too much salt, because this is common knowledge. Just please try not to over indulge.

Trans fat-

These are fats that originate in liquid form, but through a process called hydrogenation, the fats are infused with hydrogen molecules to make them become a solid form. Any time you see the ingredient section of a food, and the word "hydrogenated oil" is present, that food contains some amount of trans fat. Definitely this is something to stay away from if you are looking to get blood into your penis.

Excess sugar and high fructose corn syrup-

Eating too much sugar causes the body to release high levels of insulin. This then triggers inflammation, which then increases heart pressure and restricts blood flow.

I realize that most of you are probably now pissed off at me. I've just told you not to eat some of the best tasting foods, and I'm suggesting that you replace them with shitty food like beets and such. Listen, the object of the game is moderation. You can still indulge every now and then and the impact will be negligible. All I'm saying is let's make healthier lifestyle and eating habits in general. These things are all healthy and good for you anyways, so even if they didnt help with penile growth, it would be a smart idea to follow this eating protocol anyway. The fact that they could possibly help with penile enlargement is a major added bonus. To put it to you another way, what's more important to you...Your taste buds, or your health and your penis?

Please note: the medical information in this book is not from an actual doctor. Please consult with your physician before starting this, or any other diet, supplementation, or exercise routine. This book is not to be used as a substitute for consulting with an actual doctor.

Chapter 16

Be patient

I would like to shift gears for a minute, so to speak. The techniques outline in this book are all considered by me to be effective. You also need to realize that this is not going to happen over night. There is no way to immediately grow your penis. Growing your penis is a marathon, not a sprint. I was originally going to write a chapter of this book that detailed some quick tricks that would cause some immediate results, even if they were not permanent. When I tried to come up with effective ways to temporarily inflate the penis with some size, I could really only come up with one quick trick.

The only quick trick? Don't ejaculate for a few days before you know that someone will be seeing your penis. I'd say about 3 days before hand is a sufficient amount of time for the penis to have a temporary added volume. This is due to a couple of reasons. First off, semen is used to being discarded, so when you dont ejaculate for several days, it is backed up and can cause a swelling of the penis and testes. Also, you will probably be more aroused because you havent ejaculated for a while, so you will probably be harder and the more aroused the person is, the harder the penis gets. A hard penis is a big penis. So if you are planning a date to make love to your wife, don't masturbate for the three days prior to this date as an example.

You might be wondering why I am not incuding the penis pumps as a way of temporarily increasing the size of the penis. Well, here's the deal. I don't care for the pumps that are out there on the market. They are very inconsistent, and sometimes painful. I have mentioned several times in this book that nothing good can come from something painful. That is why I tell you in all of my techniques that if it hurts, you are doing it wrong.

So just be patient with these methods. Let them do their thing over time. I know we live in an era where everyone wants instant gratification. I get it. What I don't want to happen though, is for you to damage, or even break your dick. (Yes that can happen.) I care about you, and your penis. This is why i stress that you must be patient with all of this. Just think, if you had started this ten years ago, you would be happy right now, so think about how happy you will be in ten years. Trust me, your penis is fine until the growth kicks in.

Chapter 17

Methods that didn't work

As I mentioned at the beginning of this book, my knowledge of penile growth is extensive over many years of trial and error, to which I have weeded out all of the effective methods from the ones that didn't measure up, or even cause damage. You should feel thankful that I have taken all of the guess work out of the issue, and left you with the tried and true ways to increase length and girth. This chapter I am going to discuss some of the things I tried that Did Not work. There were countless techniques that I tried and found out to have failed, but here are just a few that stick out in my mind. Whatever you do, DO NOT try these following methods. Definitely don't do it.

Pull real hard on it. The theory behind this was if I can just pull hard enough on my penis, I will lengthen it. This method proved to be painful and not at all effective.

Hanging weights from my penis. I thought that maybe if i hung a light weight from the tip of my penis, then it would hang lower and lower each time. It was kind of an interesting theory, however, when it came down to it, it just didn't pull through as being effective.

A lengthening device using popsicle sticks and a rubber band. I thought maybe I could train my penis to be bigger if it was sticking out nice and straight at all times. Unfortunately the rubber band cut the circulation to my penis, and the popsicle sticks just gave me a splinter. If you have never had a splinter on your dick, trust me, you dont want one there. It's very painful.

Punch it till it bruises and swells up. I thought maybe it would get a little thicker if it was bruised and swollen. Kind of like when a person gets punched in the mouth and his lip swells up real big. So, I punched myself in the crotch several times hoping for it to get big and swollen. Didn't work. Just hurt.

Taqaandan. I've mentioned this earlier is the book. This is a very controversial practice where a man bends his penis almost at a 90 degree angle, until it pops. It is a very interesting feeling. Similar to cracking your knuckles. I had a looney idea that if I did this to myself, it would crack my penile tissue, freeing up more room to grow. Instead, I learned that this process can cause the penis to break in a way. It doesnt contain a bone, so it can't actually break in that sense, but the contents of the penis can still snap.

Basically, I wanted to include this section into the book so that you can realize that I am genuine. I am who i say I am. I have dedicated my life to learning about the penis, and how to increase it. I do all of this for you.

Chapter 18

Testimonial

Before I published this book, I allowed some of my long time clients to read it before it hit the shelves. Keep in mind, I'm new to the writing thing, but I'm not new to the penile coaching thing. I'd like to share a testimonial from a man who I have personally overseen for many years, and I have been his consultant and helped improve the quality of his penis. He is an author named Benji and you can find his book about Zen if you search the internet. Here's what he had to say about my book and my coaching:

The Dick Man has really outdone himself with this one! I'm not sure if the readers will truly understand the magnitude of what is going on here. He has literally put a lifetime of penis knowlege into one easy to read book. Nobody understands the male anatomy better than Dick Johnson. I would trust him with my life, and in many ways, I do.

I first came to Dick about ten years ago. I remember being called needle dick at school when i was in the showers after wrestling practice. All of the other kids used to make fun of me. Then I got a wife, and she got mad at my penis and said that I'd never be able to get her pregnant because my penis couldnt reach the parts of her vagina that it needed penetrate. I came to Dick depressed and ashamed. He told me not to worry and he told me that he had been working on a method that was going to revolutionize the way we all handle our penises. At first, I was very skeptical, but I figured, what do I have to lose? My penis was already small. How much worse could it get?

This man literally saved my life. Right now, I am proud to say that my penis is nothing to be ashamed of, it has grown quite substantially. I'm so much more confident and relaxed now. I'm no longer worried about my penis. This man is my best friend, and has been a great mentor to me. I am so much better of a person because Dick Johnson is in my life. I wouldn't trust my penis to anyone else.

Chapter 19

Conclusion

So that's about it. I really hope that you enjoyed my book. You are now on your way to the penis that you have always dreamed of. Of course, I cannot make any guarantees. Each person is different, and what works for one person might not work the same for someone else. That is why I have included these methods. I truly hope that I have inspired you. The only thing that I can assure you is this. You are enough whether or not you have a huge penis. You are not any less of a person than anyone else. This really rings true to me now. As I look back on my days of when I had a small penis, I am kind of ashamed that I spent so much time worrying about my penis size. Be proud of who you are, and be proud of your penis.

You've now completed the genius guide to penis pride. That means you are a genius. Don't change who you are. You don't have to worry about whether your penis is good enough for someone else. It is good enough for you, and my book will be with you to guide you along the way as you continue to increase your package. Remember, your penis is huge. Your penis is quality. Your penis is sufficient. Cherish your penis.